How to Understand and Deal with Anxiety

Rasha Barrage

HOW TO UNDERSTAND AND DEAL WITH ANXIETY
Copyright © 2022 by Summersdale Publishers

Originally published in the UK by Vie Books, an imprint of Summersdale Publishers, part of The Octopus Publishing Group Ltd., in 2022. First published in revised form in North America by The Experiment, LLC, in 2024.

The Experiment, LLC
220 East 23rd Street, Suite 600
New York, NY 10010-4658
theexperimentpublishing.com

This book contains the opinions and ideas of its author. It is intended to provide helpful and informative material on the subjects addressed in the book. It is sold with the understanding that the author and publisher are not engaged in rendering medical, health, or any other kind of personal professional services in the book. The author and publisher specifically disclaim all responsibility for any liability, loss, or risk—personal or otherwise—that is incurred as a consequence, directly or indirectly, of the use and application of any of the contents of this book.

The Experiment's books are available at special discounts when purchased in bulk for premiums and sales promotions as well as for fund-raising or educational use. For details, contact us at info@theexperimentpublishing.com.

Library of Congress Cataloging-in-Publication Data available upon request

ISBN 979-8-89303-020-4
Ebook ISBN 979-8-89303-021-1

Cover and text design by Summersdale Publishers

Manufactured in the United States of America

First printing September 2024

Contents

Introduction

Do you feel safe? Hopefully, the answer is yes. You can focus on these words and block out the world around you. Unfortunately, you may not always feel this way and your attention might sometimes be absorbed by something that fills you with a sense of dread, unease or imminent risk of harm.

It might be a situation that brings the possibility of change, injury or pain; it could be the risk of germs, judgment or confined spaces; or perhaps it's simply getting through another day. Whatever the cause, the sensation is one of potential danger and it is real, debilitating and all-consuming; the feeling commonly known as anxiety.

Whether you have a medical diagnosis or you suspect your worries are getting out of hand, Part 1 of this book will help you understand what anxiety is and the potential cause of your feelings. A range of tools are then outlined in Part 2 that can help you to gain a greater sense of control, safety and empowerment.

PART 1

Understanding Anxiety

Mental health disorders are widely under-reported globally and yet 284 million people were diagnosed with an anxiety disorder worldwide in 2021. Comprising almost 4 percent of the global population, it is the mental health disorder that affects the most people and it is common everywhere. But what exactly *is* anxiety?

The following pages will introduce you to the science of anxiety, what causes it and why it is so prevalent. The most common symptoms, triggers and disorders will be outlined to help you understand whether you have anxiety and explain the possible reasons why.

What is anxiety?

Anxiety is an emotional experience and it is part of what makes you human. It is a normal response designed to protect you in situations that are new, challenging or potentially threatening. As the body's protector, it is vital for your survival as it guides you between danger and safety. It is also what helps you to perform well in tests and interviews or cope in an emergency; when it is triggered, it sharpens your thoughts and puts you on "high alert."

However, your mind is not always accurate in gauging danger. The anxiety experienced can be out of proportion to the risk at hand or continue for longer periods than is necessary—this is when anxiety becomes a problem.

Fear, stress and anxiety

Fear, stress and anxiety are often confused so it's worth understanding the difference between these terms. They all relate to a threat that inspires a "fight, flight or freeze" response in your body, with important distinctions:

- Fear—this is about real-world danger. Something in the present moment is causing you to be scared for your safety or the safety of others.
- Stress—this is when you are struggling to cope with demands or expectations placed on you that can be mental (e.g., workplace) or physical (e.g., athletic training).
- Anxiety—this is about danger that is perceived in your mind but may not be accurate. It can occur in reaction to a situation that you consider stressful or frightening.

There's nothing "wrong" with you

Anxiety is part of being human. It is designed to keep you safe by preparing your body for action. Put simply, if you sense some sort of danger, to defend itself, your brain will release hormones that cause physical and mental changes. Once the danger passes, your hormone levels should return to their base level.

Given anxiety's importance in your survival, you can't make it vanish. While it is unpleasant and even debilitating at times, its absence would be much more dangerous. That's why there is no quick "fix" and you can't expect it to disappear altogether—what you can do is learn more about why you have anxiety and then take steps to mitigate it.

The science behind anxiety

Anxiety starts in the thalamus section of your brain, which is highly sensitive to information that relates to your survival. Once activated it automatically triggers the amygdala part of your brain, which deals with your reactions and activates the stress response—flooding your body with adrenaline and cortisol to sharpen your senses and quicken your reflexes. Your brain doesn't think about the danger, it simply reacts rapidly and without question, and those reactions are out of your awareness and control.

This domino effect occurs regardless of whether the trigger is from your environment (i.e. the real world) or imagery, thoughts or fantasies; your brain struggles to distinguish between what is real and what is imagined.

This means that your brain is so sensitive to threat that anxiety can be triggered by simply glancing at an image that is unsettling, or at the mere thought of something frightening. That's why just thinking about something you fear can make you feel afraid; your mind and body react even if the threat is not real.

This distortion between what is real and fake has its benefits in allowing you to be fully immersed when watching a film or listening to a story, but the downside is that your sense of threat (and your body's automatic anxious response) can be inspired by a thought or image that isn't present in real life or it can continue well past a dangerous situation.

Feeling anxious vs. having anxiety

Anxiety is a normal and necessary emotion for your survival—although the meaning of "survival" is different in the twenty-first century compared with the time of your cave-dwelling ancestors. So, if you experience some anxiety in the lead up to a specific event—such as a job interview or a speech at a wedding—and if the sensation feels proportionate to the situation and isn't affecting other parts of your life, it's likely you're experiencing "normal" anxiety.

A problem arises when the anxiety occurs on a regular basis, unexpectedly or in everyday scenarios. Perhaps you can't seem to stop yourself from worrying or you've started to avoid socializing, doing certain things or visiting certain places. If your anxiety is overwhelming or excessive to the point of affecting your quality of life, then this might indicate a problem—an anxiety disorder.

Primal fears

The cause of anxiety and anxiety disorders can be complex, but often at its core is a fear of something *imagined* in the present or future, that has developed from a *real* fear from your past. This can become clearer if you consider two primal fears that you share with all humans— namely, death and abandonment.

So, to put it simply, if you notice that your anxiety is related to present or future physical suffering, illness or pain, then this is likely to be about your (natural and highly understandable) fear of death.

If instead, your anxiety seems to arise in situations where you fear present or future rejection, humiliation or "failure," then your anxiety relates to your (equally reasonable and universal) fear of abandonment.

Why is anxiety so common?

It all comes down to survival. Your brain is the result of millions of years of human evolution, culminating in your brain's ability to automatically react and deal with threats to your survival. While those threats may no longer be a predatory animal or insufficient food to feed your tribe, danger exists in different forms: pain/illness, loneliness, unemployment, news alerts, data hacking, identity theft and so on.

The history of anxiety as a disorder is also not a recent phenomenon, though the precise terminology has changed over time. Joseph Lévy-Valensi, a French professor of psychiatry, defined *anxiété* in the early twentieth century as a "dark and distressing feeling of expectation."

Highly sensitive people

Studies have found that some brains are more sensitive than others—a trait known as "sensory processing sensitivity," which is thought to be present in an estimated 1.4 billion people globally. If you are one of these "highly sensitive people," you are more responsive to your surroundings (for better or worse), such as people's moods, strong smells, bright lights and even caffeine, and you require extra time to process information and stimuli. This heightened emotional reactivity and overstimulation also means that you are more susceptible to anxiety.

What does anxiety feel like?

The sensation of anxiety is different for everyone and it can manifest itself in your thought processes as well as physical changes.

The effects on your mind can be as follows:

- Having a sense of dread or unease
- Feeling tense and unable to relax
- Increased irritability
- Difficulty concentrating or remembering
- Needing lots of reassurance from others or feeling insecure about how others feel toward you
- Rumination (repeatedly thinking about one situation or conversation)
- Depersonalisation (feeling disconnected from your body, like you are observing yourself from the outside)
- Feeling emotionally numb during or after a stressful experience

These psychological changes are part of your mental armor, to increase your chances of survival in the face of a threat.

Physically, the effects of anxiety can include the following:

- Heavy, quick breathing
- Tension in your muscles
- Back problems
- Headaches
- Feeling dizzy
- Fidgeting and being restless
- Teeth grinding, especially during sleep
- Raised blood pressure
- Quick or irregular heartbeat
- Sweating or hot flushes
- Difficulty digesting food
- "Butterflies" in your stomach
- Feeling nauseous
- Reduced sex drive
- Sleep problems

Many of these reactions occur because they are part of preparing your body for a burst of energy, so that you are ready to fight or flee from the danger that your mind has perceived.

Can anxiety be inherited?

There is growing evidence to suggest that some people might be more susceptible to anxiety if there is a history of it in their family (known as "anxiety sensitivity"). The research is ongoing to determine whether the cause is learned behavior during childhood or genetics.

A 2021 study that looked at DNA and anxiety disorders found pioneering evidence to show locations in the human genome where variations in the sequence tend to occur in people with anxiety. This, together with other large-scale studies conducted in the preceding 20 years, suggests that anxiety may indeed be inherited.

Emotional scars

One factor that can make you more susceptible to anxiety is a highly stressful or traumatic experience in your past, particularly if it occurred when you were very young. This makes perfect sense if you remember that anxiety is your body's protector; an experience that put your life in danger or made you feel weak and vulnerable will inevitably make your brain extra sensitive to any similar situations or reminders of that experience. This could be neglect as a child, physical or emotional abuse, living through a war (or escaping one), the loss of a parent, being bullied and so on.

What triggers you?

Some experiences or environments can cause symptoms of anxiety to arise (or increase) and these situations are known as triggers or risk factors. These can be common triggers that resonate with many people, or there might be specific ones that are personal to you. Recognizing your unique, personal triggers is an important step in managing your anxiety as it gives you the opportunity to address the causes directly.

Some questions to think about are as follows:

- Is your anxiety related to certain situations, people or places?
- Are there places or environments where your anxiety has never or rarely arisen?
- Does it peak at particular times of the day?
- Are there times when your worries relate to real risks and your anxiety is a proportionate, reasonable response?

What's your problem?

Remember that the problem is not *you*; there is a certain situation in life that creates anxiety for you, so you need to identify what that problem is. It might be a constant, regular presence (maybe it's your workplace, going outside or interacting with others) or a particular issue in one location or aspect of your life (such as flying or public speaking). If you can start to understand the root cause of your anxiety, then you can avoid being self-critical and recognize what you need to change in order to deal with it effectively. This involves thinking about what might have triggered anxiety in your past (personal risk factors) as well as your present circumstances (social and environmental risk factors).

Busy, busy, busy

Stress should be a good thing. It prepares you to perform at your best in response to a particular situation (such as an interview or sports event) by ensuring you are mentally prepared and alert. However, long-term or "chronic" stress means a prolonged activation of your body's natural stress response, which can wreak havoc on your body. Chronic stress can change the chemicals in your brain that regulate cognition and mood, disrupt your sleep and circadian rhythms, and even enhance irrational fears. All this can potentially lead to you developing an anxiety disorder.

The modern world makes us all more susceptible to chronic stress. Our brains are simply not designed for the levels of information that we commonly absorb daily and the number of decisions we have to make, particularly due to the internet, smartphones and emails. For instance, when you think you are multitasking you are, in fact, just switching rapidly from one task to another and, as the neuroscientist Earl K. Miller states, there's "a cognitive cost in doing so." Your cortisol levels (i.e. stress) and adrenaline levels (fight-or-flight response) both increase, and the fuel your brain needs to focus (oxygenated glucose) is depleted. This repeated switching between tasks, and its hormonal impact impact, can naturally lead to anxiety.

Blue light

Your body has something called a "circadian clock," which synchronizes some of your biological processes through a daily cycle, partly regulated by natural daylight. The systems affected include your sleep/wake cycle, hormone release and cellular function.

If you spend a great deal of time indoors and rely on artificial light in the evenings and night (including TVs, tablets and smartphones), it is possible that your internal rhythm is being disrupted—which can make you more susceptible to anxiety. Studies show that the length and duration of exposure to artificial light (especially blue light) can reduce the quality and quantity of your sleep, which can consequently increase your anxiety levels.

Are you sitting comfortably?

Your interior surroundings, including the levels of natural light, colors, furniture and layout, can have an impact on your level of relaxation or anxiety. For instance, research at the University of Texas found that predominantly grey, beige and white office environments cause feelings of sadness and depression among employees. Think about your home or work environments and consider the following:

- Is there a persistent lack of sunlight?
- Are the ceilings low?
- Is the space cluttered?
- Are there any indoor plants or flowers?
- Is there art on the walls?

The way your home or workplace is arranged has an inevitable impact on your sense of security and comfort, which can correspondingly heighten or reduce your anxiety.

Mood and food

Nutritional psychiatry has been a growing discipline during the twenty-first century, and investigates the impact of food and supplements on mental and emotional health. Sugar, high-salt foods, alcohol, drugs, caffeine and even the amount of water you drink can impact the way you feel, including your level of anxiety. For instance, research has shown that women whose diets are high in vegetables, fruit, fish and whole grains are less likely to have anxiety disorders when compared with women who consume processed foods such as chips, pizza, white bread and soft drinks. Think about your diet and whether you consume high levels of any of the following, which have been found to raise anxiety: fruit juice or soft drinks, white bread, artificial sweeteners (aspartame), caffeine, energy drinks, alcohol and all types of processed foods such as cereals, pastries, processed meat or high-fat dairy products.

Uncertainty

Kahlil Gibran wrote, "Our anxiety does not come from thinking about the future, but from wanting to control it." If you are extra sensitive to uncertainty and tend to avoid any situations where you have to concede control, then this mindset can be a source of anxiety.

Research tells us that people vary in their ability to tolerate uncertainty. People who struggle with uncertainty often plan ahead, seek constant reassurance from others, create extensive to-do lists, avoid delegating, double (and triple) check everything and keep their calendars full. Maybe your automatic response to unpredictable situations is to worry, or you get concerned that every choice available to you is the wrong choice. When you are faced with any situation that has an uncertain outcome, then you might assume the worst, start getting anxious and believe that you are unable to cope with the worst-case scenario.

DIAGNOSING ANXIETY

Your anxiety is unique to you—stemming from your own personal history and circumstances. This is partly why it can feel incredibly lonely. Regardless of any statistics about anxiety's prevalence and commonality, the experience and fear involved is different for each individual because anxiety is unique to a person's own life story—combining genetic, developmental, environmental and psychological factors.

Bearing this in mind, there *are* features shared across some forms of anxiety, which are grouped together and known as "anxiety disorders" by medical professionals.

If you have symptoms of anxiety, you can speak to your doctor about how you're feeling and determine whether you might be showing signs of an anxiety disorder. The following pages outline the most common disorders, but there are many others.

It can be easy to gloss over statistics when it comes to matters of the mind. The knowledge that there are millions of other sufferers may provide little comfort when you feel overwhelmed with anxiety and completely alone in how you feel. But these numbers *are* significant: behind every digit is an individual with a unique experience that led them eventually to see a doctor and obtain a medical diagnosis. There is inevitably a complicated and fascinating story behind each person's anxiety, just like your own—and this might remind you that your feelings are similarly very human and normal. For instance:

- One out of every 14 people meets the criteria for an anxiety disorder.
- It is estimated that 50 percent of people suffering from anxiety are not diagnosed or adequately treated.
- In 2020 alone, 52 million women and 24 million men were diagnosed with anxiety disorders globally.

The following pages describe the most common anxiety disorders.

What keeps anxiety going?

Has your anxiety been ongoing for several years? If that's the case, then it might be worth considering your thinking patterns. Here are some reasons why your anxiety might have persisted for an extended period:

- You may have a natural tendency toward worrying and have an anxious personality.
- You may have experienced stress for a prolonged period, causing you to be in a constant state of anxiety with little to no respite.
- You may be caught in a vicious cycle of anxiety. This could be caused by either the way anxiety

feels (which can be frightening and unpleasant enough to create a fear of the symptoms of anxiety), the way you think (overestimating the danger and overlooking your ability to cope), your actions (such as avoidance, escape, alcohol or seeking reassurance) or by difficult circumstances (such as stressful relationships, work environments, unemployment, health problems etc.).

Understanding and diagnosing your anxiety will also illuminate the reasons as to why these feelings persist. Read on to learn more about the most common conditions that could be causing your anxiety.

Generalized anxiety disorder (GAD)

If you are constantly worrying and showing signs of persistent anxiety, you may be diagnosed with GAD. Perhaps you regularly wonder "what if . . . ?" and automatically envisage worst-case scenarios in everyday life, or you seem unable to relax and continually feel anxious. You worry more than most people and your fears are easily triggered, without being able to think rationally or problem-solve effectively. It is likely that you misinterpret or overestimate the risks in several situations. This will inevitably have an adverse effect on your well-being, social activities, sleep patterns and your physical health.

Panic disorder

If you regularly experience panic attacks, then your anxiety may be considered a panic disorder. Panic attacks are sudden, overwhelming sensations of fear lasting approximately 5 to 20 minutes. During a panic attack, most people experience a rapid heart rate, hyperventilation, chest pains, sweating, shaking and dizziness. The symptoms build rapidly and can be very frightening in their intensity and speed (hence the word "attack"). The sudden onset and shock can unfortunately lead to the symptoms escalating further as you can easily misinterpret them as dangerous.

A panic disorder can occur on its own or with other anxiety problems, particularly agoraphobia. Agoraphobia means a fear of leaving safe places, and the perceived danger outside could be physical, emotional or relate to other people or possessions. Sometimes the fear of having panic attacks can lead to agoraphobia.

Post-traumatic stress disorder (PTSD)

If you have experienced or witnessed a traumatic event, it is normal (and somewhat expected) to have a period of difficulty and to be plagued by memories or vivid flashbacks for a while. Some argue that it is your brain's way of trying to keep you safe and avoid it happening again. However, if you experience prolonged intrusive memories, negative mood changes, insomnia or irritability that increase over time, then you may be diagnosed with PTSD. The distress of the memories is effectively altering your behavior and may be causing you to avoid anything that might remind you of it further. Your recollections may not be visual; you may be having flashbacks of certain smells, sounds or physical sensations. You might feel fear, grief, disgust, anger or emotionally numb; a range of emotional reactions have been linked with PTSD.

Phobias

Phobias are intense fears that have grown out of proportion regarding specific objects or circumstances. Phobias can take many forms, such as arachnophobia (fear of spiders), emetophobia (fear of vomiting or seeing others being sick), haematophobia (fear of blood) or brontophobia (fear of thunder). You may have never unlearned a "built-in" fear from childhood, such as a fear of heights or strangers, or you may have developed a fear that has increased over time and steadily restricted your life (to avoid the object of fear). This can impair the quality of your life as phobias often lead to avoidance.

Social anxiety disorder

You might be diagnosed with social anxiety disorder, otherwise known as social phobia, if you excessively worry about social situations (before, after and during). The anxiety centers around how others perceive you; it relates to feeling observed or judged negatively and the risks of being seen as incompetent or doing something embarrassing. It might be a general fear of any situation where people are present, or it could be specific to certain scenarios such as eating with company or public speaking.

Because social interaction is a necessity, social anxiety disorder can be a debilitating condition that severely affects your quality of life, with an inevitable impact on your self-esteem.

The way social anxiety presents itself can vary between different cultures around the world. *Taijin kyofusho* is a form of social anxiety in Japanese and Korean cultures. This is like social anxiety disorder in terms of being concerned about social situations, but here the anxiety relates to offending, embarrassing or causing distress in *other* people rather than yourself. Rates of social anxiety disorder vary greatly between different countries and urban versus rural environments, with high rates in the US and across suburban areas worldwide.

Studies indicate that social anxiety levels may be rising due to the prevalence of social media. As sufferers retreat to the relative "comfort" of digital connection and avoid face-to-face communication, the fear of social interaction further escalates.

Obsessive-compulsive disorder (OCD)

If you regularly experience intrusive thoughts against your control, feel a need to repeatedly do certain things or focus obsessively on thoughts or images to feel safe, then you may be suffering from OCD. Do you recognize any personal habits that you feel obligated to perform in a ritualistic or special way? Perhaps you feel compelled to wash, count or organize in a particular way or adhere to some form of strict self-imposed rule. These rituals are intended to make you feel safe (from harming yourself or others) or avoid "bad luck." While you may feel short-term relief, these urges and the constant sense of obligation can easily interfere with daily life.

Body dysmorphic disorder

You may be diagnosed with body dysmorphic disorder if you feel overly anxious about your appearance and find yourself constantly worrying about your (imagined or imperceptible) physical flaws or a particular part of your body. Perhaps you spend a considerable amount of time every day applying makeup or choosing clothes, and regularly look in the mirror or avoid mirrors altogether. You may believe that you are "ugly" and frequently turn to plastic surgery or dermatologists, or perhaps your self-consciousness causes you to avoid social situations. Your preoccupation may also lead you to develop OCD, as you may start engaging in repetitive, time-consuming behaviors to manage your appearance.

Body-focused repetitive behaviors (BFRB)

If you habitually pull your hair out, bite your nails, pick at your skin or pick, pull or bite any other part of your body in a repetitive manner, then you may be suffering from a BFRB. You may not even be conscious of this behavior, or it might be an ingrained habit that briefly relieves you of your anxiety or is a form of anxiety management.

These behaviors are considered disorders as opposed to habits if they are compulsions that you find hard to resist. They may be causing you physical problems as well as emotional distress.

Eco-anxiety

Knowing about the risks of climate change, even without being adversely affected by it, has been found to cause anxiety in a rising number of people around the world. First defined in 2017 by the American Psychological Association, eco-anxiety (also known as "eco-distress" or "climate anxiety") refers to a "chronic fear of environmental doom." It is not considered a clinical condition like the other disorders described in this book, but rather a reasonable response to the very real dangers posed by global warming. It is likely to become more common during the twenty-first century as the situation worsens and media coverage increases. You may be concerned about the immediate impact of climate change (such as rising sea levels and wildfires) and/or what the future will bring for you and generations to come.

PART 2

How to Manage Anxiety

Understanding your anxiety is an important first step in dealing with it. But if you want to manage it and see a positive change in how you feel, then it's time to consider the different options available to you.

The following pages offer a series of exercises to try. Some can be done regularly and are intended to build your resilience and overall well-being so that your anxiety becomes more manageable. Others may suit a particular situation and are intended to help you cope when your anxiety arises. Most importantly, they are *ideas* that you are free to pick and mix, according to your own personal needs.

Trust yourself

If you experience anxiety, it is likely that you are overestimating a danger and underestimating your ability to cope.

As outlined previously, anxiety often stems from feeling unsafe. There is a fear of a particular situation or sensation, and this fear can be triggered by an endless range of possibilities. One way to alleviate your anxiety is to enhance your sense of safety—to start to trust either the situation you fear or the sensation you avoid (or both), as well as beginning to feel secure in your ability to manage the situation.

While it is impossible to know for certain whether something "bad" will happen, your anxiety levels will decrease if you start to habitually consider other, positive, possibilities and build trust in your ability to cope with any given scenario.

Time to refocus

Perhaps you have been grappling with anxiety for many years and the thought of ever feeling differently seems impossible. Maybe your efforts to manage it have focused entirely on the object of your fears or on the anxiety itself. Perhaps you can function, live and work day to day despite your anxiety and have avoided taking measures to address it.

If you have now reached a point where you wish to take control of your anxiety and find ways to manage the symptoms, then your attention needs to broaden to every *other* aspect of your life. What can make your life better? How can you build your sense of self-worth, well-being and vitality? The causes and triggers of anxiety are diverse; likewise, there are many choices you can make to mitigate those causes and build resilience against your triggers.

The comfort system

As discussed earlier, anxiety activates the "threat system" in your brain to prepare you for action—for fight, flight or freeze. What is perhaps less well known is that your brain also has a "comfort" or "soothing" system, which *deactivates* you and provides a sense of calm and contentment. This system releases feel-good hormones such as oxytocin and endorphins, and automatically operates when there is no threat to your safety or after a threat has passed.

As someone who suffers from anxiety, it is likely that your comfort system is underutilized or completely blocked. If you can learn ways to trigger your comfort system (through self-compassion), then your brain will automatically do its job to dial-down your levels of anxiety and increase your overall sense of safety and well-being.

Self-compassion

Research shows that your brain's comfort system can be activated through self-compassion. This means treating yourself with love, kindness, acceptance and understanding—the way you might treat a friend when they are suffering.

Self-compassion can go far beyond your anxiety, because anxiety is only a tiny part of who you are. According to Dr. Kristin Neff, self-compassion is comprised of three elements:

- Self-kindness vs. self-judgment—rather than thinking negatively about yourself and being self-critical, understand that imperfection, obstacles and failure are natural and inevitable parts of life.
- Common humanity vs. isolation—rather than feeling isolated, remember that any feelings of vulnerability, inadequacy or suffering reveal your shared humanity.
- Mindfulness vs. over-identification—allow your mind to observe and acknowledge your anxiety, but don't exaggerate it and let it define you.

If you struggle to engage in self-compassion, studies show that showing compassion toward other people equally triggers your comfort system.

The tips in the remainder of this book are essentially about putting self-compassion into practice through changes in your behavior, routines or thought patterns. Change in itself might give you a sense of anxiety or vulnerability, so be gentle with yourself. No one finds change easy, so try to be sensitive and patient with your needs.

You are likely to learn skills and adopt new, beneficial habits if you build on what you are drawn to and what you are naturally good at— don't force yourself to try something you know you won't enjoy or that might cause you greater anxiety. Do what feels right for you. This is all part of personalizing your approach to anxiety management so that it becomes entrenched in your lifestyle.

Learn to self-regulate

Have you ever felt particularly calm and exhilarated after doing some exercise, participating in a sport, or after a challenging exam or interview? Part of the reason is that you have allowed your nervous system to alternate between being settled and activated, and to regulate itself. You have triggered your fight-or-flight response and managed to calm yourself afterward.

If you start taking steps to improve your ability to self-regulate, your anxiety levels will naturally decrease. This involves recognizing that you have a choice in how you react to situations and becoming aware of your passing emotions. These states of mind can be developed through the tips in the following pages.

Haste makes waste

The word "multitasking" was first used in the 1960s to describe a computer's capability—in the twenty-first century, many people apply the word to themselves every day. Modern life can make you feel that you must be producing or always consuming and that being "busy" is a hallmark of success. Natural rhythms and body clocks have been disrupted by long working hours, 24-hour accessibility and a daily onslaught of emails, news and responsibilities.

If you rush from one thing to the next and feel a constant need to be "doing," then this frenetic pace of life is likely to be adding to your anxiety. By slowing down, you can learn to simply "be." As Ruby Wax wrote in *A Mindfulness Guide for the Frazzled*, "We need to wake up and notice the signals that our minds and bodies are giving us; to slow down sometimes and notice the scenery."

Grounding

When you are overwhelmed or slightly anxious, grounding techniques can help you to feel instantly calmer, reassured and in control. These can refocus your thoughts and stop your anxious feelings from escalating further. Here are some techniques you can try:

- Simply stand with both feet on the floor, shoulder-width apart. Place all your awareness on the bottom of your feet and any sensations you can feel.
- If you're sitting, move your bottom to the back of the chair and focus on its textures and material. Push your feet into the ground and imagine a color floating through every part of your body, starting with your head and down to your toes.
- Hold an object in your hand and give it your full attention. Consider its weight, color, patterns and texture.
- Place one hand over the crown of your head and close your eyes.

Laugh it off

Laughter feels good for many reasons, including the fact that it induces physical changes in your body that can alleviate anxiety. When your muscles move and tense as you laugh, your intake of oxygen increases and endorphins are released in your brain. Endorphins are the hormones that help you feel happier and calmer. Laughter also activates then quickly disables your stress response (increasing then decreasing your heart and breathing rates), giving you a relaxed feeling. The more regularly you laugh, the greater the long-term effects you will feel, including a reduction in corisol levels, boosted immune system and improved mood.

Take the time to watch your favorite comedians or sitcoms, laugh with friends, be silly with any young children in your life, try laughter therapy— think of what makes you laugh and make that a regular part of your routine.

Rest and digest

The vagus nerve is a long nerve connecting your brain to your heart, lungs and stomach. It signals your body to relax after experiencing anxiety (or any stressful situation), by decreasing your breathing and heart rate and activating digestion. If your vagus nerve isn't functioning adequately or loses its resilience, this can lead to a heightened stress response, which can develop into anxiety.

Because the vagus nerve works in tandem with your breath and heart, you can improve its functioning by learning to control and manipulate your breath—which, in turn, automatically affects your heart rate. Put simply, your breath tells your heart how fast it should beat, and your heart rate tells your vagus nerve whether to rest and digest (or not). By engaging in breath work, you can effectively "tone" your vagus nerve and mitigate your symptoms of anxiety.

23,000 breaths a day

The way you breathe, both normally and during stressful times, could be causing or exacerbating your anxiety.

When you are in a state of stress or anxiety, it is likely that you breathe at a rapid pace through your mouth. This fast, shallow breathing causes your brain to believe that you are in a danger- ous environment, triggering your sympathetic nervous system and putting you on high alert— whether for a brief period or for days and weeks at a time (including disruption to your sleep). The breathing expert Patrick McKeown has described this as a "feedback loop," where your anxiety causes you to breathe faster and the faster breathing feeds further anxiety.

By slowing down your breathing, you can calm your state of mind and reduce your anxiety levels. As Dr. Rangan Chatterjee says: "Breathing is information. The way you breathe is the way you live."

To improve the way you breathe, there are several techniques you can try. Here are two to get you started:

- 4-7-8 deep breathing—close your mouth and breathe in through your nose to the count of 4, hold your breath to the count of 7 and release your breath to the count of 8. Repeat 2 or 3 times to avoid getting lightheaded.
- Deep belly breathing—place a hand on your stomach and the other on your chest. Take slow deep breaths in through your nose to fill your stomach with air. Control your breath so that you notice your stomach inflating while your chest stays still.

The most important thing is to slow and lengthen your exhalation. This will engage your parasympathetic nervous system (which includes your vagus nerve) and make you feel calmer and more relaxed.

Meditate

Studies show that regular meditation can reduce stress, lower blood pressure and ease anxiety. There are many ways to meditate, including breath awareness, body scanning or the repetition of a mantra. Some meditation techniques are intended to alter your attitude while others are to release tension or encourage mindfulness. Regardless of your personality or lifestyle, there is likely to be a form of meditation that suits your needs. You can try guided meditations (some relate directly to anxiety), which are available via apps and online, or attend a group meditation practice in your area.

If you have never tried it before, you can start by simply finding a quiet place where there are no distractions and gently closing your eyes. For a few minutes, focus your attention on the rise and fall of your breath and if thoughts arise, just let them pass without dwelling on them and without judgment, returning to the breath.

Stop

To practice meditation, you have to hit "pause" on your life and make time to do it. Unlike mindfulness exercises, which you can practice in any situation, meditation can provide a welcome break from your day-to-day routine and encourages you to prioritize stillness and relaxation. It also prevents you from compulsively dwelling on past experiences or future worries, and allows you to be at peace in the present moment.

Thích Nhất Hạnh described it in his book *Fear*:

> *You stop totally in the present moment. And when you stop, you are master of your body and mind. . . . Sitting meditation is not for fighting. You let go of everything.*

Compassion for others

Anxiety can cause you to focus on yourself and the struggles you are facing. A powerful way to counter this is to actively care for others. Studies show that engaging in acts of kindness and compassion can increase your sense of happiness, optimism and satisfaction. You could check in on friends, family and loved ones, or take time to engage in volunteer work. Providing support to others can broaden your perspective, helping you to see beyond your anxiety or to view your situation in a more positive light. Self-esteem can also be boosted through helping others, which is important to help you approach and overcome anxiety-inducing situations.

Starfish up!

One of the most powerful tools for managing anxiety also happens to be the quickest and most accessible—your posture. As mentioned in Part 1, research shows that your levels of confidence and relaxation are not only the result of your mindset but also your hormone levels. In particular, high amounts of cortisol increase your levels of anxiety and reduce your ability to cope with stress. Testosterone increases confidence and therefore your ability to cope with pressure. One way you can adjust these hormone levels is by simply changing your body language so that you expand your physical presence.

Studies show that expansive, powerful poses can reduce your cortisol levels by 25 percent and increase your testosterone levels by 20 percent. If you become more aware of your posture, you can start adjusting it throughout your day to regulate your hormone levels accordingly.

In her book, *Presence,* Amy Cuddy talks of the Wonder Woman "power pose" (which is not restricted to women), whereby you stand tall with your hands on your hips and your chest out. You could try this before any situation that typically induces your anxiety, or again as a regular daily practice for 1 to 2 minutes to adjust your hormone levels. Another way to remember this is using the phrase "starfish up!" Another way to remember this is using the phrase "starfish up!" to describe stretching your body out like a starfish, perhaps as part of your morning routine or before a potentially stressful situation.

Try to consistently pay attention to posture, particularly on occasions when you feel the onset of anxiety. The optimal body position is as follows:

- Back straight
- Chest open
- Shoulders back
- Legs/arms uncrossed
- Standing/sitting tall

Look after your neck

If you spend hours every day driving or looking at your smartphone, tablet or computer, you might unconsciously adapt the way you sit and stand. Perhaps you position your head forward and bend your neck, causing your shoulders to also bend downward (known as "tech neck"). This exaggerates the curve of your spine and causes your body to curl inward. You may also experience strain in your hands or elbows due to constantly gripping your smartphone (known as "text claw"). These types of positions can increase stress, lower self-esteem, lower assertiveness and increase your anxiety. To minimize this harm, you could reduce the time you spend driving, opt for larger devices or screens, try postural therapy (such as the Egoscue method), see a chiropractor or do exercises that strengthen the muscles in your core, shoulders and neck.

Move your body

Engaging in any form of exercise provides a multitude of benefits that can help to alleviate your anxiety, such as:

- Reducing cortisol levels (the stress hormone)
- Reducing muscle tension
- Releasing endorphins, which lower your perception of pain and trigger a euphoric feeling in your body. By boosting your mood, you can feel more positive and capable.
- Boosting self-esteem and providing a sense of mastery; important for trusting yourself to handle anxiety-inducing situations
- Improving sleep, which helps to manage anxiety

Exercise also replicates some of the physical symptoms of anxiety: fast heart rate, sweating and breathlessness. By inviting these sensations, you can be assured that they are temporary, and not dangerous. This makes you less likely to panic the next time you experience anxiety symptoms.

Rhythmic movement has also been shown to help alleviate anxiety. If you engage in activities that require you to move your body from left to right (such as walking, running or dancing), you also stimulate your brain from left to right. Research shows that moving your body repeatedly in a rhythmic way can help to reduce the distress you feel about something and hence help you to process and make sense of an event. You can therefore view situations that cause you anxiety in a more objective way, from a calmer reflective mindset.

If you're short on time, focus on your core. Studies have shown that your stomach muscles are directly connected to your adrenal glands (which produce a variety of hormones including adrenaline and cortisol), so you can decrease your stress response by strengthening these muscles.

Runner's high

Studies show that running can be an extremely powerful tool for both the prevention and management of anxiety symptoms. Just one running session increases blood flow and oxygen to the prefrontal cortex in your brain, which improves your decision-making abilities and reduces impulsivity. Running on a regular basis also increases your attention span. This greater mental clarity can help to ease your anxiety and make you feel less overwhelmed. The immediate sensation of the strength and power in your body can also boost your self-esteem. Aside from the physical benefits, the ritual of running is significant in itself because it is an act of self-care and prioritization. If you dislike running or it is impractical for you, then regular brisk walks can provide many of the same benefits.

Seek connection

Loneliness can be an inevitable consequence of anxiety. A 2021 study that measured social interactions using real-time data through an app found that people who exhibited high stress levels one day tended to have less social contact the following day—something that had only previously been seen in animal studies. This occurred regardless of gender or personality. This inclination to withdraw when we are stressed could have an evolutionary purpose; it may have served as an effective survival strategy for our ancestors when fleeing from predators, but, as described in Part 1 of this book, your brain does not distinguish between perceived and real dangers. If your anxiety is causing you to feel lonely and isolated, then you could try taking control of the matter and contacting someone you trust—even a short message could start a conversation and create a sense of connection.

Find your support circle

Researchers have found that social support is a protective factor against stressful life events. Your anxiety is likely to come and go throughout your life, so it's important to be comfortable with that knowledge and to build a supportive group of people around you that you will always feel comfortable discussing your feelings with. Your vulnerability to anxiety will decrease with a greater number of social connections, particularly if you have friends to confide in. Sharing your worries and challenges can be cathartic and provide welcome relief if you are struggling. This is part of helping you to process what is happening, as well as allowing you to gain some perspective and reflect on your experiences. Think about who you can talk to, or people who can distract you from your feelings when that is what you need.

Online support forums

There are numerous anxiety support groups online, where you can talk openly with people who will be able to understand and relate to your anxiety. You can participate anonymously if you wish and share your innermost thoughts, safe in the knowledge that you will not be judged or misunderstood. If you are not sure where to find one, you can search for forums that are run by or in connection with mental health charities. These also have the benefit of being moderated, so the conversation will be respectful and genuine.

Deep muscle relaxation

If you spend any time with three- or four-year-olds, you will know that relaxation does not come naturally and is a skill like any other. You need time to learn how to relax, even as an adult. This skill is vital because you cannot feel anxious if you are in a state of relaxation. If you have anxiety, your body is not relaxed and your muscles are in a state of tension.

One method that could help to reduce your overall levels of anxiety is known as "deep muscle relaxation," which you can practice daily and start to use in everyday situations. This requires you to progressively tense groups of muscles as you breathe in and then relax them as you breathe out.

As you tense your muscles, study the tension for a few seconds and then relax them. A slight tingling sensation means the muscles are relaxing.

Choose a time of day when you feel the least anxious, then lie down, close your eyes and follow a tense/relax cycle with the following groups of muscles (in order):

1. Hands—clench, then relax.
2. Arms—bend your elbows and tense, then relax.
3. Neck—tilt your head back and slowly roll it from side to side, then straighten your neck into a comfortable position.
4. Face—lower eyebrows in a frown then relax your forehead, or raise your eyebrows, then relax. Clench your jaw, then relax. Close eyes tightly, then open gently.
5. Chest—take a deep breath and hold it for 4 to 10 seconds, then relax.
6. Stomach—suck it in tightly, then relax.
7. Bottom—squeeze tightly together, then relax.
8. Legs—straighten your legs and point your toes toward your face. Then point your toes away and wriggle them.

Strike a pose

Yoga is an ancient Indian practice containing many of the elements that help to manage anxiety, such as breath regulation, mindfulness, reframing your thoughts and concentration. As a form of exercise that combines relaxation, meditation, stretching and breathing, it can increase your awareness of the link between your mind and body while also reducing your stress hormone levels. A study in 2020 found that yoga was significantly more effective at improving symptoms of generalized anxiety disorder than stress management techniques.

There are many types of yoga you can try, including hatha (which involves gently holding poses and focused breathing), satyananda (which involves deep relaxation and meditation) and power yoga (which emphasizes movement through poses). You could start with just a few poses, which you can find many examples of online, such as child's pose, savasana, forward bend and downward-facing dog, or attend a yoga class in your local area.

Try qigong

Qigong (pronounced *CHEE-gong*) is a branch of traditional Chinese medicine that involves coordinated breathing, meditation and gentle, fluid body movements with the aim of building and balancing your qi—translated as "life energy."

If you find that deep-breathing exercises have a positive impact on how you feel, you could try combining this with the slow, rhythmic body movements and stretches involved in qigong. It is relatively easy to learn and practice, and you may find that the combination has a more profound effect and helps to reduce your anxiety further.

The power of touch

One way to relieve your anxiety is by having a massage. Massage therapy has been found to ease physical tension, aid relaxation and promote your overall well-being. There are more subtle benefits too; the sensation of physical touch can be incredibly grounding and help to draw your attention away from your anxious thoughts and into your body instead. If a registered practitioner or loved one is not available to give you a massage, then a self-massage—on your shoulders, hands or feet—can provide some of the same benefits.

Dim the lights

Exposure to different types of light may influence your anxiety levels. Studies show that artificial sources of blue light such as fluorescent light and LED lighting can have an effect on the human body—a key finding when you consider the worldwide dominance of such lighting in workplaces, hospitals and schools, as well as your phone, computer and television. Research shows that this type of lighting makes you more alert, consequently reducing your ability to relax and negatively impacting sleep; factors that are not conducive to alleviating anxiety (especially panic disorders). You might notice an improvement in your anxiety levels by minimizing screen time and bright lights during evening hours and increasing your exposure to natural light in the daytime and energy-efficient bulbs that emit "warm light" or "soft light" instead.

Sleep better

Sleeping difficulties are frequently linked with anxiety, as both a symptom and a trigger. If you are suffering from anxiety and in a state of mental hyperarousal, this can prevent you from falling asleep easily. Even after you fall asleep, you might find yourself waking up in the middle of the night, and you struggle to fall back asleep as your mind is filled with worries or stress. If you are sleep deprived, this can cause you to feel anxious or heighten your existing anxiety. Due to this cyclical relationship between anxiety and sleep, building healthy sleep habits to ensure better rest can be a vital tool to help you manage your anxiety. Fortunately, there are many tried-and-tested ways you can improve your sleep.

The following techniques have been recommended by the neuroscientist Dr. Matthew Walker, to increase the quantity and quality of your sleep:

- Create a daily sleep routine that is maintained during weekends. Leave time to unwind before bed and always go to bed at roughly the same time.
- Avoid intensive exercise 3 hours before bed.
- Reduce your caffeine or nicotine intake.
- Reduce alcohol and other drinks. Alcohol impairs your "deep sleep" and your ability to breathe well at night, which can cause you to wake up several times. Try to avoid any fluids for the 2 hours preceding bedtime, to avoid waking for bathroom trips.
- Avoid eating meals 3 hours before bed (to prevent indigestion, which interferes with sleep).
- Your bedroom should resemble a prehistoric cave and be gadget-free, cool and dark. Do not sleep with your phone nearby.

Stay hydrated

Dehydration impacts more than just the function of your body; it affects your mood and emotional state and can even heighten your anxiety. An easy and pleasant way to look after yourself and remove one potential trigger is to simply drink more water.

To know whether you are drinking enough, you can look at the color of your urine, which should be pale. Aim for 6 to 8 glasses of water per day (about 2 liters); a target that is easily achievable if you always carry a reusable bottle. You could also set alarms or reminders on your phone. The important thing is not to wait until you feel thirsty, but to drink consistently throughout the day.

Keep calm and drink (herbal) tea

Humans have been drinking herbal tea for centuries—and for good reason. As well as their pleasant taste and scent, they can provide a range of health benefits including improved sleep, reduced blood pressure and anxiety relief. There are countless options for you to try, with studies showing the following to be particularly helpful for anxiety: chamomile, peppermint, green (decaffeinated), lavender, kava, rose and ginseng tea, as well as teas that include lemon balm extract, ashwagandha, gotu kola, passionflower or turmeric. You could drink one (or a combination) of these herbal teas when you feel particularly stressed or anxious, or as a routine complementary therapy.

Reduce your stimulants

If you often turn to coffee, tea, cigarettes or chocolate when you are stressed, their short-term comfort comes at a price. These stimulants release adrenaline in your body, which heightens symptoms of anxiety. Alcohol also becomes a stimulant when it is metabolized, increasing your feelings of stress. There are additional consequences of all these stimulants, including disturbed sleep and fatigue. As a very general guide, adults should limit caffeine to 14 fluid ounces (400 ml) per day (about four cupfuls of coffee) and alcohol to one or two drinks per day (with at least two alcohol-free days per week). Research shows that caffeine consumed 6 hours before bed can impair the quality of your sleep. If used as long-term coping strategies, then addiction, ill-health or excessive weight could add to your anxiety. Avoiding or limiting these items from your diet could leave you feeling healthier and less anxious.

Brighten up your food

Studies have found that people who eat less than three portions of fruit and vegetables a day are more likely to have an anxiety disorder compared with people whose diets are rich in fruit and vegetables. One theory is that low fruit and vegetable intake can lead to weight gain, which may, in turn, increase systemic inflammation. Inflammation has been found to impact brain function and trigger symptoms of anxiety.

If you think your diet may be affecting the way you feel, you could try increasing your intake of fruit and vegetables. Eating more of the following foods has also been found to reduce anxiety: Brazil nuts, dark chocolate, eggs, oily fish (which is high in omega-3), pumpkin seeds, turmeric, yogurt containing "friendly" bacteria and fermented food (such as sauerkraut and kimchi).

Boost your vitamins

Research suggests that various supplements, including omega-3 and several vitamins, can help to relieve the symptoms of anxiety. Think about your diet or any supplements you have and consider increasing your intake of B vitamins (particularly B-12), magnesium, L-theanine or simple multivitamins. Vitamin D deficiency has also been linked with anxiety disorders. You can get more vitamin D through increasing your sun exposure or eating foods such as salmon or mackerel. If you follow a vegetarian or vegan diet, then vitamin D supplements can be taken instead.

To look after your brain health, you can increase your intake of omega-3 fatty acids (or take supplements if your doctor approves it), which is found in some oily fish and flaxseed.

Reduce sugar

Studies show that consuming food that is high in sugar can trigger anxiety or heighten anxiety symptoms, as well as reducing your body's ability to cope with stress. This is because high-sugar food causes your blood sugar to spike and drop faster than food that is not high in sugar. If your blood-sugar level quickly spikes then drops, this will directly impact your mood and exacerbate your anxiety. If you suffer from panic attacks, there is the added possibility of misinterpreting some of the physical sensations of a sugar rush as signs of an impending attack, therefore causing greater anxiety. To combat this, you can try to reduce your sugar intake and start eating more food that is low in sugar and high in fiber.

Calming scents

The scents from essential oils derived from plants can be a surprising—and highly pleasant—way to alleviate stress and anxiety. For instance, studies have found that the calming smells in essential oils from cedar trees can lower stress hormone levels. This is because the airborne odor molecules interact with all your body's organs that relate to smell, including the limbic system in your brain (commonly referred to as the "emotional brain"). There are numerous options you can try, including lavender, chamomile, orange, sandalwood, clary sage, rose and jasmine.

They can be diffused (e.g., through reed diffusers or candles) or applied topically when diluted, and some can be directly inhaled with a drop or two on a cotton ball or tissue. Just bear in mind that essential oils are highly concentrated and can cause allergic reactions. They should be used in moderation and with caution, according to the instructions provided.

Draw tech boundaries

Increased phone usage has been directly linked with anxiety, particularly when it includes a large amount of time reading negative news stories and comments. The term "doomscrolling" entered the Oxford English Dictionary in 2020, but the compulsive drive to search for answers when we feel anxious or afraid is not new. Research shows that overexposure to bad news stories can cause hyperactivation (thus increasing your anxiety) or immediate numbness followed by insomnia or nightmares.

Here are some ideas you can try to remain informed while also reducing your screen time:

- Check the news just once a day, preferably in the evening.
- Remove all banner-style/sound notifications from your phone.
- Avoid going online if the reasons stem from boredom or anxiety.
- Vow to be away from your phone for an hour every day, or even a full day.
- Keep your phone out of sight when socializing.

- When commuting, avoid looking at a screen and try listening to podcasts, audiobooks or music.

Social media has been found to have a detrimental effect on both mental and physical health. It can create anxiety about a fear of missing out (FOMO) or lead you to constantly compare yourself to the image being presented by other people, adding to anxiety regarding your appearance, lifestyle, popularity and so on. Studies have found that the harmful effects even apply to people who are socially isolated.

To avoid passive scrolling, you could uninstall social media apps from your phone or deactivate accounts one by one to see if there is a noticeable difference in how you feel. Deactivating accounts has been shown to have a positive effect in reducing anxiety. If you continue using social media, research shows that you can minimize its potential harm by limiting your use to 10 minutes per platform per day (used actively rather than passively, with a clear intention at the outset).

Get creative

Engaging in creative activities has been extensively proven to relieve both stress and anxiety. This is because creativity causes your brain to release large quantities of endorphins, serotonin and dopamine—all chemicals that induce feelings of pleasure and satisfaction. When you focus entirely on the act of creating and cause these changes in your brain activity, you can enter a "flow state" (as coined by psychologist Mihaly Csikszentmihalyi) that is similar to the experience of yoga, mindfulness and meditation. If an activity is challenging and/or fun, connectivity in the brain also increases, which improves emotional resilience.

The beneficial effects of creativity occur during the *process* of creation; the result is somewhat irrelevant. So, lack of talent, skill or experience should not prevent you from trying something creative, whether it is art, music, dance, film, or anything else that sparks your curiosity.

Morning pages

In Julia Cameron's seminal book, *The Artist's Way*, the pivotal tool to unblock and release creativity is said to be three pages of "longhand, stream of consciousness writing" first thing in the morning. One benefit of this exercise (which she named "morning pages") is that it releases your negativity on to the page, so those thoughts no longer cloud your day. While this is directed toward unblocking creativity (which is an additional benefit for anxiety purposes), you may find that practicing morning pages helps to diminish your negative thoughts, clear your mind and improve your self-awareness—all important steps for reducing anxiety. To try this, have some paper to hand and simply write three pages shortly after you wake up. Put down every thought that occurs to you—without pause, correction or judgment—and then repeat for as many days as you wish. Come back to the process when you find your anxious thoughts are building up again.

Rewire your brain

If you sometimes despair that your anxiety will remain the same or think that you have no power to alter how you feel, then it's important to be aware of your innate capacity for change. Since the moment you were born until today, your brain has been constantly forming new connections and pathways and rewiring itself to meet your evolving needs—an ability known as "neuroplasticity." You can literally rewire your neural pathways and change the chemicals in your brain, including those that increase or decrease your anxiety.

Studies show that enriched environments (saturated with novelty, focused attention and challenge) are critical for promoting neuroplasticity, such as travelling, learning a musical instrument, creating artwork, dancing and reading fiction. By trying any of the activities suggested in Part 2 of this book, you are effectively taking action to rewire your anxious brain.

De-centering or psychological distancing

One way to prevent and alleviate symptoms of anxiety is by shifting your perspective and taking an objective viewpoint on negative thoughts and feelings. To achieve this, you need to actively create time in your day to process what's happening and clarify your thoughts. This will help you to notice the feelings you're having and simply sit with them, allow them to pass and recognize that they are temporary. Trying to ignore or deny your anxiety will not make it go away; taking a few minutes to just acknowledge and accept it is an important step toward managing it.

Think of RAIN

One way to improve your ability to handle anxious feelings is by using something known as the RAIN technique, as coined by Tara Brach in her book *Radical Acceptance*. This is achieved the following:

- Recognize when you feel anxious.
- Acknowledge, accept and allow your anxiety to exist, without trying to fix or avoid it.
- Investigate your feelings. Ask yourself why. Can you identify the cause of your feelings?
- Non-identification with the feelings—this means you know that the anxiety does not define you; it is a passing feeling and not permanent.

Correct thinking mistakes

Your anxiety can be partly driven by distorted thinking. For instance, you might tend to exaggerate, over-generalize or have unrealistic standards. These thought habits, known as "biased thinking," can be useful for avoiding danger in certain scenarios, but they become unhelpful and anxiety-inducing if you consistently view things this way or if this type of thinking is too easily triggered. Consider whether any of the following thinking biases seem familiar to you:

- Exaggerating likelihood—do you focus on negatives and risks?
- Over-generalizing—similar to exaggerating, perhaps you draw negative conclusions from brief, small events.
- Catastrophizing—do you always assume the worst will happen? This is particularly common if you have anxiety regarding your (or someone else's) state of health.
- Absolutist thinking—do you see everything in all-or-nothing terms?

- Unrealistic standards—do you put a great deal of pressure on yourself to be perfect and to never make a mistake?
- Ignoring the positive—often dismissing compliments or reassuring facts and focusing on the negatives instead.
- Scanning—actively searching for hazards and danger in particular scenarios.
- False intuition—do you often jump to conclusions based on your impulsive reactions rather than weighing the facts?
- Self-blame—being self-critical and blaming yourself when bad things happen. Do you often take things personally?
- Worrying—filling the future with fear and constantly asking "what if?"

If any of these thinking patterns seem relevant to you, considering when this occurs might help you to understand why your anxiety increases at times. By becoming more conscious of your thought patterns, you can start to notice when your thoughts are not useful, reliable or true.

Start a thought diary

When you are in a state of calm, it can be difficult to recall the cause of a previous spike in anxiety. To find out your triggers, it can be helpful to record your thoughts or mental images in writing at the time that you start to feel tense or show symptoms of anxiety. This may seem difficult at first, but it should become easier with practice.

By keeping a diary or log of your thoughts, you might also notice the amount of "biased thinking" you apply, which will help you to see whether it's in proportion to the risks or threats you envisage. Ask yourself: Am I exaggerating or jumping to conclusions? Am I dwelling on the negatives? With time, you may be able to start catching your anxious thoughts and reconsidering them with something more balanced.

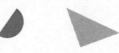

Let happiness find you

The word "happiness" derives from "hap," which means chance or good luck in Middle English. Its meaning changed over time to become a purpose in itself and, for some, it is the primary objective in life. If this rings true for you, then you might need to reconsider your perspective. As Ruth Whippman, author of *The Pursuit of Happiness and Why it's Making Us Anxious* says, the search for happiness is making anxiety worse for many people: "Like an attractive man, it seems the more actively happiness is pursued, the more it refuses to call and starts avoiding you at parties." The US, where the "pursuit of happiness" is a culturally embedded ideal, regularly claims the highest number of anxiety sufferers in the world. Try to think of happiness as a potential by-product of experiences rather than an end goal.

A perfect problem

The pursuit of perfection is often seen as a positive trait; one that exemplifies ambition and hard work. If you find that you often use words such as "should," you likely seek perfection and have unrealistic expectations of yourself and others. It's fine to try your best and have high standards, but applying excessive pressure to never make a mistake can lead to reduced confidence and greater anxiety.

Wabi-sabi has no direct translation in English, but it roughly means "perfectly imperfect" in Japanese; that beauty can be found in imperfection or flaws. Part of learning to deal with your anxiety involves adopting a *wabi-sabi* mindset instead of pessimism and struggle. Make peace with the inevitability of change and imperfection, in both yourself and the world around you. Rather than wishing for things to change or dwelling on negatives, try to notice beauty and joy throughout your day.

Exposure

Every time you have felt anxiety in the past and consequently avoided the situation, place or object that triggered it, your brain has increased your anxiety about that source of fear. This increased anxiety then leads to more avoidance and then a vicious cycle ensues.

An important step in learning to manage your anxiety is to face the things you fear. This process is called "exposure," and involves gradually and repeatedly confronting the source of your anxiety until you become desensitized to it. You can do this with the aid of a professional, through exposure therapy, or you can try practicing this yourself if you feel ready.

You could create an "exposure hierarchy." Think about one situation that causes you anxiety and break it down into eight to ten steps. For instance, if your anxiety relates to social occasions, different steps might include meeting two friends, then three friends, then attending a small dinner party, and so on until the final step of a wedding or other large social gathering.

Choose an easier activity to begin with and persist with it; try to continue past the point when you feel uncomfortable and start to feel anxious. Sitting with your anxiety for a reasonable amount of time (perhaps 10 minutes) will allow you to see that you are safe and your anxiety will start to naturally decrease. Your brain will learn that this situation is not dangerous. You could then try a slightly more challenging activity and repeat the process.

It's OK to feel anxious

If you are only willing to expose yourself to the situations, places or objects that you fear *until* you start to feel anxious, then you will not effectively deal with your anxiety.

Know that your fear will not disappear—so make the conscious decision that you want to take control of your anxiety and that this is more important than avoiding your fear. You can use mindfulness techniques to accept and feel your anxiety in the moment without an urge to escape from those uncomfortable feelings.

For exposure to be effective, it's important to do the thing you fear while you're afraid so you will know that your fear is a false alarm and that you are not in real danger.

Worry time

One technique you can try is to set yourself a convenient time every day as "worry time." This means allowing 20 to 30 minutes of uninterrupted time to write about everything that is worrying you. This focused time could be spent trying to solve some of your problems, or simply acknowledging your feelings and concerns without any pressure to find a solution. During the rest of the day, when you notice your anxiety rising or your mind worrying, you can tell yourself that you can focus on this during your "worry time" (and only then), allowing your thoughts to shift back to the present.

Positive thinking

Practicing optimism can help reduce anxiety, and the way to encourage this is through positive self-talk. One simple exercise developed by the psychologist Barbara Fredrickson is to pause, look around and ask yourself, "What is going right for me right now?" Another idea by Mel Robbins is to high-five your reflection in the mirror every morning or whenever you need reassurance, because your brain and nervous system are hardwired to associate high-fives with positivity. By improving your ability to spot the positive things in your life, you will also be in a better position to celebrate those positives. Research suggests that gratitude alone may not reduce your anxiety, but overwhelming evidence shows its power to improve your self-esteem, relationships, sleep, and even your brain and biological functioning. You could try keeping a gratitude journal or regularly expressing your thanks to family, friends or people you appreciate.

Distraction

If you sense your anxiety developing, one way to stop its escalation is through distraction. Your mind can only really focus on one thing at a time (despite your best efforts to multitask), so instead of thinking about the trigger for your anxiety, or perhaps the anxious feelings themselves, try concentrating on something else. Here are some distraction techniques you might want to try:

- Fidgeting, such as playing with candy wrappers, stress balls or putty—this hugely underrated method can be enough to absorb your attention and reduce your stress
- Doodling
- Reciting a poem
- Planning your next holiday or day off
- Organizing, tidying or cleaning
- Physical activity or exercise

Find a technique that works for you; make sure it involves thoughts or activities that you enjoy and that require your full attention. Distraction can hopefully stop your usual cycle of thoughts from spiralling into uncontrollable anxiety.

Problem-solving techniques

A lack of trust in yourself might underlie some of your anxiety. An important way to boost your self-confidence is to change how you perceive challenges and opportunities in life; events that might seem negative (like job loss, relationship breakdowns, etc.) can actually prove to be opportunities for you to recognize your ability to cope; you can get through these things and survive. This self-awareness can help you to approach anxiety-inducing situations with less trepidation and greater confidence in yourself. As Susan Jeffers wrote in *Feel the Fear and Do It Anyway*, "Security is not having things; it's handling things. Thus, when you can answer all your 'what ifs' with 'I can handle it '... the fear disappears."

A study by Harvard University shows that it takes less effort for the brain to jump from anxiety to excitement than anxiety to calm. So next time you feel anxious, you could try telling yourself that you are excited instead. This form of "anxiety reappraisal" may not make you less anxious, but it will help you to perceive opportunities rather than obstacles.

You could try setting goals for yourself (many of the tips in this book can be used to help you). Goals can be helpful because setting them implies that things can be different, and that change is possible. Goals also shift your focus on to possibility rather than difficulty—providing a sense of hope that can carry you through times of heightened anxiety.

Make space

If you are often surrounded by cluttered surfaces or drawers and cupboards that are full and disorganized, then this could be adding to your feelings of anxiety. If the idea of decluttering seems overwhelming, you could try just setting aside 10 minutes to organize a drawer or sort one shelf. Disposing of unwanted clothes or possessions can also be quite a cathartic process, helping to clear your mind as well as your living space. *The Happiness Project*'s Gretchen Rubin recommends making your bed every day, without exception, as a means of maintaining outer order.

Watch your words

The words you use when you communicate your feelings can affect your anxiety. If you use positive, empowering words then you acknowledge your ability to handle yourself, whereas the use of negative, helpless words will leave you feeling vulnerable or unable to cope in relation to the same situation. For instance, replace "I can't" with "I won't" and "I should" with "I could," so you recognize that you have a choice regarding your actions. Any inconvenience or unfortunate event is best described as a "learning opportunity." These may seem like petty semantics, but the repetition of positive versus negative words can reinforce how you feel about yourself and your ability to cope with anything that comes up in life, including situations that cause you anxiety. As psychologist Susan Jeffers said, "Not only does your sense of yourself change with a more powerful vocabulary, so also does your presence in the world."

N-O is O-K

Many of us struggle with the word "no," and take on far too many tasks and projects without considering whether it's in our best interests. If you feel that you are overloaded with duties and responsibilities, and that this is adding to your anxiety, try to resist your urge to say "yes" next time someone asks you for a favor or for additional work that is beyond your capacity. Consider delegating or outsourcing any of your tasks and try to set boundaries on your time and effort. In addition to the quantity of work you have, consider your attitude to its *quality*; do you constantly seek perfection or do you acknowledge when "good" is "good enough"? For trivial tasks, you can avoid perfectionism by simply asking yourself whether there is any real benefit in spending more time and energy on it.

Embrace uncertainty

Research shows that people vary in their ability to tolerate uncertainty. If you struggle with uncertainty and tend to plan and control as much as you can, then this may be adding to your anxiety levels. You might find it helpful to become more accepting of uncertainty as an inevitable part of life. You could try to change your behavior to act as if you are comfortable with it. For instance, you can start to plan less, be more spontaneous and delegate more. Don't spend too much time looking at all the options or potential outcomes of minor decisions. Let other people be in control and coordinate things for you. Building your tolerance for uncertainty may be difficult at first—and out of your comfort zone—but with time you may find that it helps to alleviate your anxiety.

The power of now

Anxiety can put your thoughts squarely into the past or future: there is a sense of dread or fear about a perceived threat, and the anxiety is likely to have developed from past experiences and avoidance. By exercising mindfulness, you can train your brain to start being more present in the moment and observe your thoughts (including those causing you anxiety). When you feel anxious, mindfulness allows you to acknowledge your emotions without them overpowering you. Instead, you learn to sit with your feelings, pay them attention in a calm, detached way and then let them pass. As Jon Kabat-Zinn says:

> *Mindfulness is about being fully awake in our lives. It is about perceiving the exquisite vividness of each moment. We also gain immediate access to our own powerful inner resources for insight, transformation and healing.*

Mindfulness techniques

If you struggle to calm your thoughts and get into a state of relaxation, then you may find that mindfulness techniques can help. As Thích Nhất Hạnh stated in his book *Fear*, the practice of mindfulness is the practice of coming back to the here and now to be deeply in touch with ourselves and with life. We have to train ourselves to do this.

One way to start is to find a quiet space without distractions and a few minutes to yourself. Take the time to slow down your breathing and become aware of your surroundings—think about the emotions passing through you, your body, the sights and smells around you.

If thoughts pop up that relate to the future or other things concerning you, that's fine—accept the ebb and flow of your thoughts and bring your mind back to the present sensations you can see, hear, feel, smell and touch.

When you practice mindfulness, you can take it with you wherever you go. If you start to feel anxious or before you enter a situation that you know causes you stress, exercising mindfulness can provide you with a sense of safety and confidence. As the Buddhist monk Haemin Sunim teaches, "When the mind looks outward, it is swayed by the heavy winds of the world. But when the mind faces inward, we can find our center and rest in stillness."

Write a haiku

If you find it difficult to simply "be" and feel the urge to always "do," then one way around this is to practice writing a haiku. A haiku is a short form of poetry originally from Japan. It consists of 3 lines and up to 17 syllables, with a common structure of 5-7-5 syllables. A haiku does not need to rhyme and, most importantly for anxiety purposes, the traditional focus is on natural imagery, seasons and the here and now. Here is an example from the seventeenth century by Matsuo Bashō:

A field of cotton
As if the moon
Had flowered

Writing a haiku can awaken your senses and allow you to be more mindful, in an unforced way. You can start by taking a notebook and sitting somewhere quiet outside, such as a garden or park, or pause on a countryside walk. Write down what you see, feel, smell and hear, and then try shaping some of the words into a haiku.

Your inner child

If you struggle to be kind to yourself and to exercise self-compassion, one technique to overcome this is to picture yourself as a child (or perhaps a child in your life that you are close to). Imagine that the child is anxious their parents are going to separate, they're being bullied at school, they are lost in a busy street or distressed for any reason. Which soothing words would you say? How would you treat this child? Linger with these thoughts for a few minutes and allow this exercise to gently steer you toward greater self-compassion. Showing compassion for others is also proven to trigger the comfort system in your brain, releasing oxytocin and endorphins, which leads to a reduction in your anxiety levels.

Seek awe-inspiring experiences

When you encounter a sight that is epic and wondrous, your heart rate and blood pressure drop. It can also give you a different perspective on life. Awe can be found anywhere, but key components can be novelty or physical vastness. Research has found that weekly 15-minute "awe-walks" can cause increased positive emotions and less distress after only eight weeks, and increased exposure to awe-inspiring moments can make you more generous and cooperative. A University of California study found that inducing awe may relieve the worry of waiting for uncertain news, and that you can experience this sense of wonder through listening to beautiful music or watching a deeply affecting film.

Look at fractals

Your physical surroundings can potentially reduce your levels of anxiety. Experiments using MRI techniques have found that the human brain is "hardwired" to respond to complex forms in nature that repeat at different scales, known as "fractal patterns." Some examples are trees, clouds, coastlines, snowflakes, pinecones, rivers, or spirals in plants and animals.

Studies show that exposure to fractal patterns can reduce your levels of stress by as much as 60 percent. Patients in hospitals have also been found to recover more quickly if their windows look out to nature. If you live or work in an urban area, a similar effect can be achieved by viewing art that replicates these patterns, such as nature photography, Islamic art or paintings by artists like Jackson Pollock. According to physicist Richard Taylor, even a short period spent looking at such patterns can induce a state of "relaxed wakefulness."

Green time

Nature employs the mind without fatigue and yet enlivens it. Tranquilizes it and enlivens it. And thus, through the influences of the mind over body, gives the effect of refreshing rest and reinvigoration to the whole system.

This was said by the American landscape architect Frederick Law Olmsted in the nineteenth century and science is starting to confirm it. Nature's numerous benefits include the following:

- Sights—people living near trees have better "amygdala integrity," meaning a brain structure that can cope better with stress. Some researchers argue that you have an innate, genetic affinity to nature, so your senses and body rhythms are attuned to the natural world (known as the biophilia theory).
- Sounds—there is reduced tension in the nervous systems of people listening to birdsong. The sound of cars and airplanes increases tension.
- Smells—trees, particularly coniferous trees, emit essential oils called phytoncides that activate your immune system.

You may have heard of the Japanese therapeutic practice known as *Shinrin-yoku*, meaning "forest bathing." This refers to a complete immersion in a forest atmosphere to reap its numerous benefits for your health. It is achieved by walking, running or cycling in a forest (or any vast green space) and consciously connecting yourself to the nature around you with all your senses, through your eyes, ears, nose, mouth, hands and feet. Studies have shown its numerous health benefits, including improved concentration, higher pain thresholds and reductions in stress, blood pressure and heart rate. Research has found that spending time near water can have a similar effect (termed "blue mind" by author Wallace J. Nichols), whether that involves walking on a beach, sailing on a boat, swimming or scuba diving.

According to Dr. Qing Li, you can set yourself in the right frame of mind for forest bathing by taking a few simple steps:

- Leave your phone at home.
- Take it slowly and forget about the time.
- Find a place to sit.
- Notice what you see and hear.
- Stay for 2 hours (though benefits can be felt after 20 minutes).

Seek silence

Do you experience moments of silence during the day? If not, then this might be contributing to your feelings of anxiety. Excessive noise can make you more stressed and increase your cortisol levels.

While you might assume that silence heightens anxious thoughts and worries, studies show the opposite effect. Being in quiet environments has many health benefits, including reducing cortisol levels, lowering blood pressure and encouraging mindfulness. Even slow, relaxing music does not have the same positive impact on your heart rate and blood pressure as complete silence.

Here are some ways you can create more silence in your day:

- Turn off background music.
- Reduce the use of headphones or earbuds.
- Use breaks from work as opportunities for silence.
- Wake up extra early while the rest of the world is still sleeping.

Ask for help

"What is the bravest thing you've ever said?" asked the boy. "Help," said the horse. "Asking for help isn't giving up," said the horse. "It's refusing to give up."

This quote is from Charlie Mackesy's *The Boy, the Mole, the Fox and the Horse* and it perfectly captures the courage needed by all of us when we decide to ask for help. There can be a multitude of reasons to avoid asking for help. You might not want to be a "burden," or believe that you will be perceived as weak, vulnerable or incompetent. You may also fear rejection or handing control over to someone else.

If you have kept your anxiety hidden from others, opening up to someone may prove to be a huge relief. The reaction may be supportive, concerned or surprised; what matters most is taking that first step to share your feelings and ask for help.

MEDICAL TREATMENTS

If you have tried several of the ideas and techniques set out in this book but find that you are still struggling with your anxiety, then it may be time to seek professional support.

Speak to your doctor and be completely honest about how you are feeling so they can diagnose the form of anxiety you have and offer you the most appropriate treatment. They might offer you psychological treatment (such as cognitive behavioral therapy) and/or medication, depending on your physical and psychological symptoms. Your doctor can prescribe a variety of different types of medication, which can either be for short- or long-term use. The medication options include antidepressants, anticonvulsants or sedatives (for short-term use in severe cases). Your doctor should be happy to discuss what each of these do and cover any possible side effects; don't be afraid to ask questions. The different therapies you might be offered are outlined in the following pages.

Talking therapy

Your source of anxiety can be caused by a range of factors that are unique and personal to you. With so many factors involved, it's no surprise that there are a range of different anxiety disorders that suit varied treatments. For instance, if you suffer from social anxiety disorder, your needs will differ from someone who suffers from panic attacks. Because of this, therapy can be an effective treatment as it treats more than just the symptoms of the problem (which is the limitation of anxiety medication).

A therapist is someone who can apply research-based techniques to help you overcome your difficulties and develop more effective habits. They can help you to identify the causes of your anxiety and learn tools and coping mechanisms that are tailored to your specific needs.

The length of therapy will depend on the type and severity of your anxiety, though many are short-term courses of treatment. According to the American Psychological Association, eight to ten therapy sessions are usually sufficient.

If in-person therapy is too costly or inconvenient for you, online or telephone therapy may be available. You might find that therapy sessions held from the comfort of your own home can help you to speak openly and honestly about your issues.

Of the various types of therapy available, the most common ones used for anxiety are cognitive behavioral therapy and exposure therapy.

Cognitive behavioral therapy (CBT)

CBT is a practical form of therapy that focuses on your present rather than your past. It aims to help you identify your thinking patterns and gain a greater understanding of how your thoughts, behaviors, feelings and emotions are intertwined. It teaches you to recognize that your negative thoughts are just thoughts and not facts, and how to replace them with more positive, balanced thinking. The key benefit of this form of therapy is that it recognizes *you* as the expert of your own experiences and empowers you to identify the tools and techniques that serve you best. The therapist does not give you all the answers or direct your behavior, they simply collaborate with you to identify the steps you can take to create change. It has been proven to be an effective treatment for many people suffering from anxiety.

Exposure therapy

Exposure therapy encourages you to gradually confront the object of your anxiety, to build your confidence and learn coping strategies. It involves a step-by-step approach, usually with a gentle start, in a setting that is only mildly threatening, and then developing from there (a process known as "systematic desensitization"). This form of therapy can be effective in breaking the cycle of avoidance and fear, which is a common trait in all forms of anxiety. The pace and type of exposure can also vary depending on the best strategy for you; it might be direct, imagined or through virtual reality technology. Research shows that exposure through virtual reality can allow you to gain familiarity over time if gradual, physical exposure is not possible. For instance, if your anxiety relates to flying, you could take a virtual flight in the therapist's office that replicates the sights and sounds of a real airplane.

Eye-movement therapy

There is a theory that emotional torment and unprocessed memories from your past (for instance, abandonment by a parent) can trigger anxiety in the present. This is because your brain can react in the same way as if that earlier experience is being repeated (for instance, always fearing abandonment by a partner). If you suspect that this applies to you, then one method you might like to try is eye-movement desensitization and reprocessing therapy (EMDR). This requires you to discuss those traumatic experiences while a therapist directs your eye movements. This can reduce the pain attached to that memory and consequently reduce your anxiety levels. It is often used for post-traumatic stress disorder (PTSD).

Counseling

Counseling is a unique form of therapy whereby the counselor does not necessarily offer you advice. Their job is simply to listen to you, without judgment, while you share your feelings, worries and thoughts. There are two types of counseling available: directive and non-directive. Directive counseling involves the counselor playing a more active role in directing the process and providing explanations, interpretations and advice where relevant. With non-directive counseling, the direction of the sessions comes from you, the client. You are encouraged to analyse your difficulties, strengths and potential solutions with the assistance of the counselor. Whichever method of counseling you choose, you might find that this freedom to "vent" and talk openly about how you feel is exactly what you need to identify the causes of your anxiety or to find the best ways for you to deal with it.

Alternative therapies

If you find that treatments or conventional talking therapies are not reducing your anxiety, or you want to experiment with different options, you can always try complementary and alternative therapies. These typically look at your physical and mental health as a whole, rather than treating them separately. Many are rooted in ancient philosophies that predate modern medicine.

Even if these alternative forms of therapy do not prove beneficial to you in the long term, you might find that they provide immediate relief and a calming effect if that is what you seek.

There are a wide variety of options, so it would be worthwhile doing some research to identify what you think will suit you best. You may wish to consider some of the following alternative therapies:

- Aromatherapy—this is where essential oils are used to rebalance the body and mind.

- Hypnotherapy—this puts you in a state of deep relaxation to access your subconscious thoughts. It may help with unwanted or repetitive thought patterns.

- Reiki or energy healing—this is a Japanese technique that involves the transfer of "universal energy" from a Reiki practitioner to you, to encourage healing and relaxation.

- Traditional Chinese medicine—this includes acupuncture, tui na (a form of massage) and herbal remedies that aim to rebalance the body's energy systems.

- Ayurvedic medicine—based on ancient Indian theory, this uses medicines made from plants and minerals to restore balance in the body. It also includes massage and panchakarma (a detoxification treatment).

Step up, or leap forward

Conventional wisdom tells you to approach anything new or challenging slowly, with a "step-by-step" approach. Perhaps you believe you should only try meditation once your work schedule eases up, or that daily exercise might be enough to reduce your anxiety to a manageable level. While these actions are a step in the right direction, studies show that you are more likely to see improvements and feel healthier, stronger and more resilient by making two or more simultaneous changes in your life. Think about the ideas presented in Part 2 of this book and, if you feel ready, try adopting a few of them at the same time, particularly if they support one another (such as reduced screen time and paying attention to your posture). Dare to leap—you might just find that overhauling several little things is what you need to see big improvements in how you feel.

Conclusion

In 1884, the philosopher Søren Kierkegaard stated, "Learning to know anxiety is an adventure which every man has to affront.... He therefore who has learned rightly to be in anxiety has learned the most important thing." So, what is the most important thing? While the answer may depend on your own unique experience, the array of tools and exercises presented in this book show that, in the face of anxiety, you remain safe from harm and, ultimately, capable. Dealing with anxiety involves thinking less about the anxiety itself, and focusing more on your own resilience, potential and possibility. At any given moment, the power to feel and live differently is always within you. All you have to do is put that knowledge into action.

Also available in the How to Understand and Deal series

Trade Paperback Originals • $9.95 US | $12.95 CAN

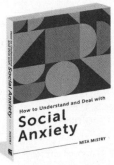

979-8-89303-024-2

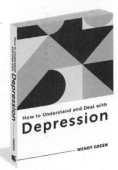

979-8-89303-022-8

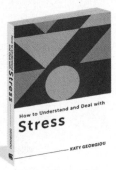

979-8-89303-026-6